GALLBLADDER DISEASE

EASILY EXPLAINED BY A SURGEON

Maria Azizian, M.D., FACS

Copyright © 2022 Maria Azizian.

All rights reserved. This book or any portion thereof may not be reproduced or used in any manner whatsoever without the express written permission of the publisher except for the use of brief quotations in a book review.

Table of Contents

Introduction	1
Chapter 1 – Facts and Statistics	3
Chapter 2 – Anatomy of Gallbladder	5
Chapter 3 – What does the Gallbladder Do?	7
Chapter 4 – What Makes the Gallbladder Sick? Overview of Gallstones & More	9
Chapter 5 – What Causes Gallstones?	14
Chapter 6 – Symptoms of Gallbladder Disease	19
Chapter 7 – Cholecystitis	26
Chapter 8 – How is the Gallbladder Disease Diagnosed? Bloodwork and Imaging	32
Chapter 9 – Surgery for Gallbladder Removal: Cholecystectomy	34
Chapter 10 – What Can Go Wrong? Risks and Complications	37
Chapter 11 – What Happens After Surgery? Post-Operative Course	40
Chapter 12 – What Really Happens with the GI System After Cholecystectomy?	42
Chapter 13 – Diet After Gallbladder Surgery	44

Chapter 14 – Special Situations: Choledocholithiasis and Cholangitis or When Gallstones Obstruct Common Bile Duct (CBD) ... 46

Chapter 15 – Special Situations: Gallstone Pancreatitis or When Gallstones Obstruct Pancreas ... 50

Chapter 16 – Special Situations: Gallstone Ileus or When Gallstones Obstruct Small Bowel ... 52

Chapter 17 – Special Situations: Gallbladder Disease When There Are No Gallstones at all ... 55

Chapter 18 – Special Situations: Slow Gallbladder ... 59

Chapter 19 – Growths in Gallbladder ... 61

Conclusion ... 63

References ... 64

About the Author ... 66

Introduction

Gallbladder disease has become an epidemic in many Western countries. In some regions, the number of surgeries for gallbladder disease has even surpassed the number of appendectomies.

Although many cases of gallbladder disease are straightforward, and treated with an algorithm- like approach, there are also variations that make this condition quite interesting.

As a surgeon, when I schedule a gallbladder operation, the pre-operative discussion and the informed signed consent state that to treat this condition, I will need to remove the gallbladder. The same scenario plays out in Massachusetts or in California or in Michigan, as removal of the gallbladder is the standard of care for a patient whose gallbladder is diseased.

Patients and their families have a lot of questions about gallbladder surgery as they try to understand what lies ahead of them.

The fundamental question I receive from patients is, "will I be okay after losing an organ, and how will the rest of my life be affected?"

Although gallbladder removal is the best option for many patients, I hope that the future of medicine will one day bring an effective treatment for this condition that will allow doctors to either cure or prevent this disease, rather than remove an organ due its malfunction.

Indeed, although some non-surgical ways of addressing gallbladder disease are being introduced (in the form of certain medications), their efficacy has yet to be established. As a result, gallbladder removal is at present the standard of care for most gallbladder problems.

This short review is for patients, their families, medical students and anyone who is curious about the amazing workings of the human body.

CHAPTER 1

Facts and Statistics

Surgery for gallbladder removal is called laparoscopic cholecystectomy, and it is the most common non-gynecological abdominal surgery performed in the United States. The number of cholecystectomies performed annually in this country is over 300,000.

Most common cause of gallbladder disease is related to the presence of gallstones.

Although approximately 20 million people in the US have gallstones, many of them do not require surgery.

The incidence of gallstones increases with age.

Women are more likely than men to form gallstones.

By age fifty-five 50% of women and 5% of men have gallstones. Surgical removal of the gallbladder is the mainstream treatment for gallbladder disease.

The gallbladder could be removed via a large open scar of several inches (open) or through 3 or 4 small scars (laparoscopic).

The standard of care in the US, as well as in many other countries, has been a laparoscopic cholecystectomy since the early 1990s.

Laparoscopic cholecystectomy was first performed by a German surgeon Dr. Mühe in 1985.

This surgery is usually performed by a general surgeon.

Most gallbladder related conditions are related to its infection and inflammation, as well, as to the presence of the gallstones. Gallbladder cancer is very rare, and in many cases has a poor prognosis.

CHAPTER 2

Anatomy of Gallbladder

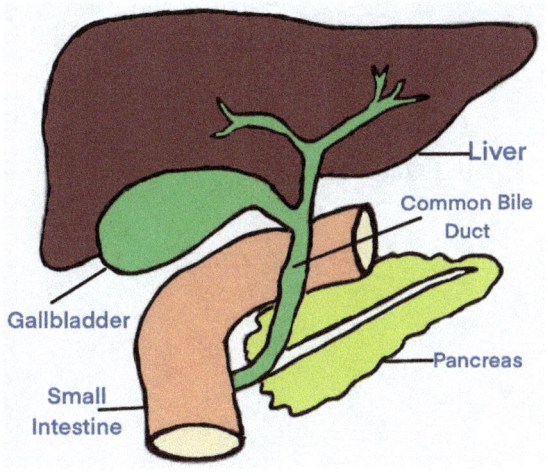

Gallbladder (GB) is a part of the gastrointestinal tract (GI). It is a small sack-like organ with an average size of a small egg. It may triple in size when infected. GB is located in the right upper abdomen on the lower surface of the liver. Often, GB is shown as hanging from the liver, but it is not completely accurate. Normal GB is attached to the liver by a thin flimsy tissue. When GB is diseased, this flimsy tissue becomes very thick and, at times, hard for a surgeon to dissect through.

Gallbladder is closely associated with several ducts, such as cystic duct, common bile duct, common hepatic duct and right and left hepatic ducts.

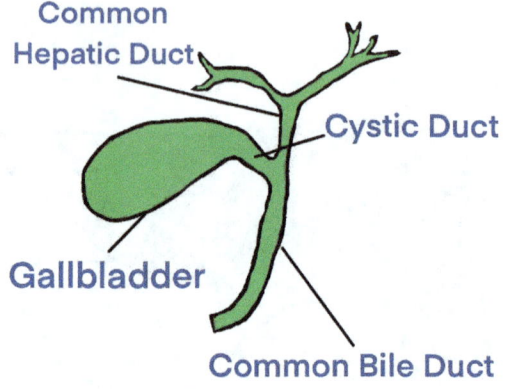

CHAPTER 3

What does the Gallbladder Do?

GB stores bile. Of note, it doesn't make bile. The bile is made by the liver.
So, first, it is a storage organ.
It also concentrates bile.
Then it ejects bile into intestine in response to food.
Additionally, GB may modify components of bile.

So how does it work in reality?
You eat a Big Mac, and, as it travels down your gastrointestinal tract, the GB contracts, and ejects bile that ends up in the small intestine. The bile breaks down the fats in the meat, mayo, etc.

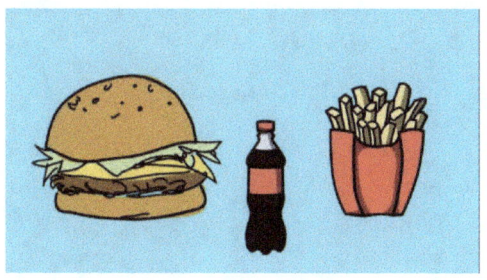

Yes, that is why very fatty foods are common triggers for the gallbladder disease. They overstrain GB, by making it work harder. It is ok in your 20s, but by the time you are 40, your poor GB may not be able to deal with daily fat-laden fast-food diet.

Wait a second, does it mean that fat is bad for you, and you should avoid fatty meals to keep your GB healthy?

Well, not so fast. This brings us to our next topic

CHAPTER 4

What Makes the Gallbladder Sick? Overview of Gallstones & More

This chapter introduces several topics that will be explored in more depth later in this book.

The most common initiating factor for the gallbladder disease is the presence of gallstones.

Gallstones look like little pebbles or, occasionally, like a brown/golden sludge.

75% of gallstones are composed of cholesterol, and appropriately called Cholesterol Gallstones.

25% of gallstones are composed of elements, such as calcium, phosphate, carbonate, and other. They are called Pigment Gallstones.

The presence of gallstones inside the gallbladder without an infection is called CHOLELITHIASIS.

When gallbladder with gallstones gets infected, this disease is called CHOLECYSTITIS.

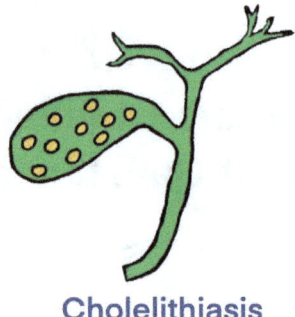

Cholelithiasis

The gallstones are not always stationary, as they may migrate to other organs and obstruct them, leading to inflammation and infection of those organs.

For example, obstruction of the Common Bile Duct with gallstones results in a condition called CHOLEDOCHOLITHIASIS.

When choledocholithiasis gets infected, it is called CHOLANGITIS.

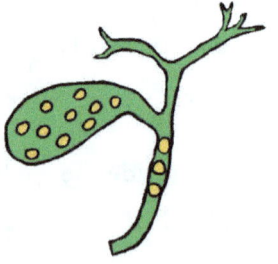

Choledocholithiasis

When a gallstone obstructs the major pancreatic duct of pancreas, it causes obstruction of the flow of pancreatic enzymes and leads to pancreatitis. Inflammation +/- infection of the pancreas due to the obstruction by a gallstone is called GALLSTONE PANCREATITIS.

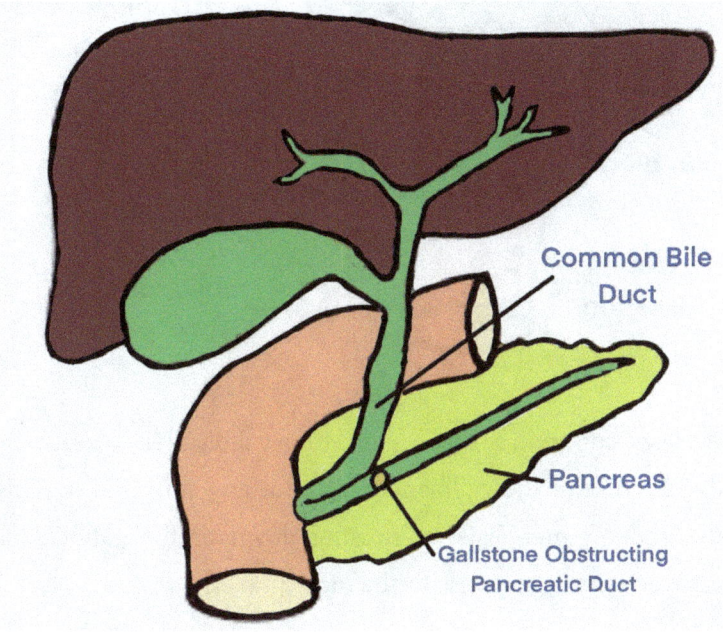

Rarely, a gallstone may get very large (sometimes the size of a golf ball or even larger), and then erode into the small intestine, causing intestinal (bowel) obstruction. This intestinal blockage is called GALLSTONE ILEUS.

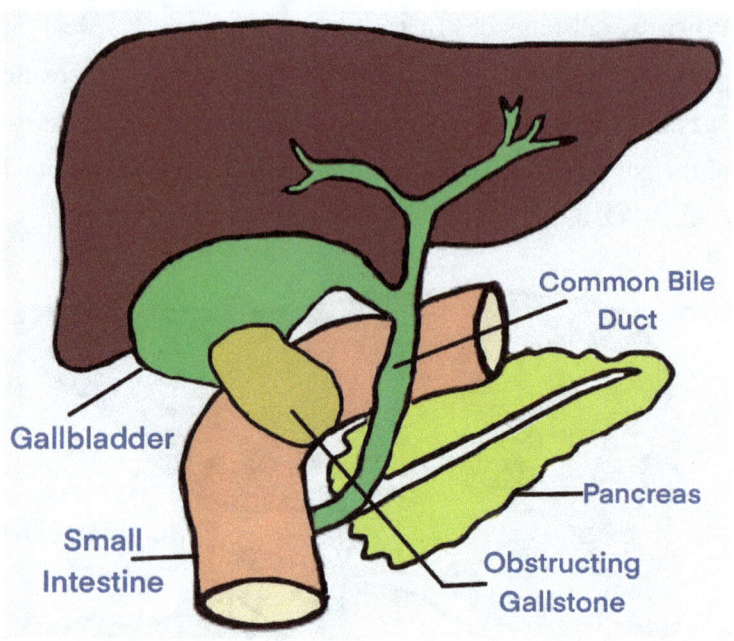

A less common reason for the gallbladder disease is dysfunction of the gallbladder without any stones in it. This dysfunction manifests as slowing down of the gallbladder contractions in response to the food intake.

In addition, there may be benign (non-cancerous) and malignant (cancerous) growths in the gallbladder.
GALLBLADDER POLYPS are benign and small growths. Unless they are growing, there is no need for any treatment or surgeries due to their presence.

GALLBLADDER CANCER is uncommon, but, unfortunately, may not be detected in time. Due to frequent absence of the symptoms in early gallbladder cancer, by the time it is diagnosed, the prognosis is not good.

CHAPTER 5

What Causes Gallstones?

Since the most common cause of the gallbladder disease, at least in the Western world, is related to gallstones, this question should be rephrased from WHAT CAUSES THE GALLBLADDER DISEASE into WHAT CAUSES THE GALLSTONES?
There are 2 major types of stones: cholesterol and pigment.

Most gallstones seen in the Western World are CHOLESTEROL gallstones.

WHAT PREDISPOSES TO THE FORMATION OF CHOLESTEROL GALLSTONES?

Female Sex
Advanced Age
Obesity
Being Inactive / Lack of Exercise
Pregnancy

The mechanism of the cholesterol gallstone formation is multifactorial, with some of the contributing factors being the following:

If bile contains too much bilirubin.

If bile contains too much cholesterol- yes, it is THE DIETARY cholesterol from the Whopper that overwhelms the gallbladder.

If the gallbladder doesn't contract properly, and unable to properly or fully eject bile.

HOWEVER, IT IS NOT ONLY ABOUT FAT AND CHOLESTEROL!

There is a correlation between an intake of simple carbohydrates and the gallstone formation, meaning drinking slushies and coke will affect your gallbladder too!

WHAT DIETARY FACTORS CONTRIBUTE TO THE FORMATION OF CHOLESTEROL GALLSTONES?

Highly refined sugars and sweets
High fructose
Low fiber
Low vitamin C intake
High fat
Frequent fatty meals
High meat consumption

It is important to note that not all fats are the same. Studies have shown that men following a diet high in monounsaturated or polyunsaturated fats were 18% less likely to develop gallstones.

Alternatively, following a diet rich in fish, vegetable proteins, fruit, and vitamin C has shown to have a preventative value in terms of the cholesterol stone formation. Olive oil has significant health benefits for liver and gallbladder, in general.

A LITTLE BIT ABOUT FAT:
Fats that are solid at room temperature are called SATURATED FATS.

SATURATED FATS ARE IN
Red meat
Coconut Oil
Processed meats: hot dogs, sausage, bacon
Packaged and Processed foods like supermarket cookies, chips
Whole (full fat) milk and dairy made with whole milk

Fats that are liquid at room temperature are called UNSATURATED.
UNSATURATED FATS ARE IN
Oils: Olive, avocado, grapeseed, sunflower
Fish: salmon, tuna
Nuts, such as almonds, hazelnuts, and pecans

SYMPTOMS FROM GALLSTONES

Pain caused by gallstones in the gallbladder is called biliary colic.

The right upper abdominal pain from biliary colic is one of the most common conditions that is presented to the emergency room (ER).

BILIARY COLIC

Scenario:

Jennifer is a 45-year-old mother of three. She is moderately overweight, has mild high blood pressure, and loves occasional trip to Burger King. She started having pain in her right upper abdomen shortly after she finished dinner that consisted of steak and mashed potatoes with gravy.

The pain was both sharp and somewhat dull at the same time. She felt sick to her stomach and vomited twice. She also started having some discomfort in her right shoulder blade. This is not the first time she has been getting these pains. They have been going on for about 2 years, and usually would come either at the end of the meal or a little after. However, the pain has never been this bad. She finally was able to go to sleep at 3 am, only to wake up at 5 am.

The pain was getting to be more intense, and she called 911. When she was seen in the Emergency Room, all her bloodwork was normal. The only finding was the presence of gallstones in the gallbladder on an ultrasound exam. After a few hours of monitoring, the pain was gone. She was discharged home and was referred to a surgeon to follow up with within a month to schedule an elective gallbladder surgery.

Although it is called biliary colic, the pain is often not colicky, but steady and dull.
Classically, the pain starts 30 min or so after eating a fatty meal. It may last up to 6 hours.
In some cases, the pain starts at night, and may wake one up from sleep.
The pain doesn't get better with lying down or passing flatus or having a bowel movement.

Question: I ate 3 burgers at 7 pm and now I have pain in my right abdomen.
Why does this pain occur?

Answer: The high fat content of burgers makes GB work extra hard via hormonal and neural (nerve) response. As it keeps contracting, some stones obstruct GB exit, meaning that the bile is trapped in GB. This leads to an increase in intra-gallbladder pressure. The increase in pressure leads to pain. As GB relaxes, the stones move away from the exit, and the bile can flow out into intestine.

Seeds, such a pumpkin, chia and sunflower
Avocados
Yes, unsaturated fats are healthier and better for you.
It is recommended by the American Heart Association that the intake of saturated fat stays at 5-6% of daily calories.
A diet high in saturated fats may lead to an increase in cholesterol and "bad fat" called LDL. In addition to leading to gallstone formation, this diet is a major causative factor in heart disease, high blood pressure, stroke, etc.

Meanwhile, unsaturated fats are good for the body, including the heart.
Unsaturated fats include MONOunsaturated and POLYunsaturated fats.
The POLYunsaturated fats are very important as the human body can't produce them, and needs to extract them from the external sources, such as fatty fish, walnuts, flaxseeds, etc.

WHAT ABOUT PIGMENT GALLSTONES?

Pigment gallstones are dark brown or black stones that consist of calcium slats of bilirubin, phosphate, and other salts. In general, they are more predominant in the Asian countries. Interestingly, there is a difference in the etiology of black and brown pigment gallstones.

Black stones are formed in non-infected bile of patients with liver cirrhosis, alcoholism, pancreatitis, and in patients who have been receiving intravenous nutrition. They are also more common in the elderly.

Brown stones are associated with infected bile, and they tend to cause more trouble as they often migrate outside of the gallbladder and obstruct other organs/ ducts.

It is interesting that gallstones could recur or form again in the Common Bile Duct after the gallbladder is removed.

> *Question: I had my gallbladder removed 2 years ago, and recently developed abdominal pain and jaundice. My doctor ordered an MRI that showed stones in one of my ducts (Common Bile Duct).*
>
> *Answer: Unfortunately, gallstones could appear after the gallbladder removal, and cause problems, just the same. In this situation the stones were formed after surgery and, subsequently, they led to an obstruction of the bile flow in the common bile duct. Thankfully, this situation is rare, and can easily be remedied with an endoscopic (through the mouth) technique of removal of the stones called ERCP (more about it later).*

CHAPTER 6

Symptoms of Gallbladder Disease

We discussed that gallstones are the manifestation of poor diet and inability of our GI tract to keep up with it, but how do they mechanically cause the disease?

As noted earlier, the gallbladder is a storage organ. The bile flows from the gallbladder and through the cystic duct into the common bile duct and, ultimately, into the small intestine.

When the gallstones are mobile and the entrance to the cystic duct is open and non-obstructed, then it is unlikely that these gallstones will cause any symptoms.

However, if the gallstones periodically obstruct and close the entrance to the cystic duct, then the patient may feel pain/symptoms during these periods of obstruction.

If the gallstones block the cystic duct and become immobile, then obstruction of a bile outflow, along with the resultant bacterial overgrowth, will lead to an infection, that may develop into a full-blown sepsis in some cases.

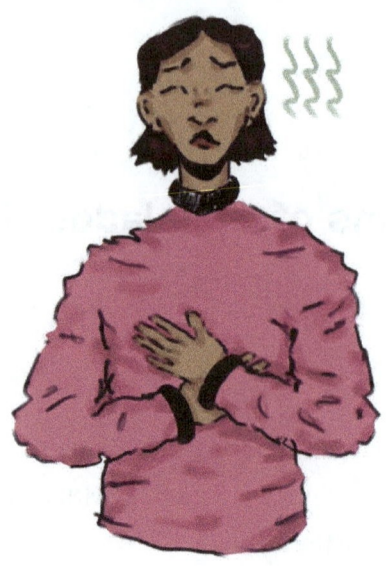

Presence of gallstones in GB without any obstruction of the cystic duct, and in the absence of the actual disease of the gallbladder, is called CHOLELITHIASIS.

Presence of gallstones in GB with infection and inflammation of the gallbladder is called CHOLECYSTITIS.

Cholecystitis with gallstones is called CALCULOUS CHOLECYSTITIS
Cholecystitis without gallstones is ACALCULOUS CHOLECYSTITIS.
Yes, another name for gallstones is calculi.

Common Symptoms of Biliary Colic

Pain in right shoulder blade
Mid upper abdominal pain
Nausea and vomiting

Uncommon Symptoms of Biliary Colic

Belching and regurgitation
Fullness of meals /early satiety
Abdominal bloating
Burning in the mid upper abdomen
Chest pain
Non-specific abdominal pain

The uncommon symptoms may be very confusing, and lead to an "over" workup in the ER. For example, a 60-year-old woman with chest pain due to biliary colic will end up getting two workups, to rule out a heart attack and to look for gastrointestinal causes of her pain. Since a heart attack is more life-threatening, a cardiac workup is initiated first. Only after it is ruled out, then gastrointestinal workup is initiated, although some tests may be happening concomitantly.

A patient with biliary colic may suffer at home or end up going to the ER.

In the ER the diagnosis of biliary colic is made when this patient has an abdominal pain with normal vital signs and bloodwork, and the only abnormal finding is gallstones.

Subsequently, it is very rare for this type of a patient with an only finding of gallstones to be admitted and / or have surgery that night. Nowadays, most commonly this patient will be observed in the ER until the pain is gone, and then sent home with instructions to follow up with a surgeon to undergo laparoscopic cholecystectomy in a near future.

The episodes of biliary colic may be sporadic or daily. In most cases, these patients end up having their gallbladder removed.

GALLSTONES AFTER WEIGHT LOSS

Question: I had a gastric bypass surgery and lost 80 lbs. in 4 months. However, recently I started having abdominal pain, and was diagnosed with biliary colic and gallstones. I thought that it is the weight gain and obesity that usually cause the gallbladder disease.

Answer: True, in most cases it is an unhealthy diet and obesity that lead to the formation of gallstones, and the gallbladder disease.
Interestingly, rapid weight loss, regardless of the method; whether due to strict dieting or weight-loss surgery, is also

> *associated with the formation of gallstones. For that reason, it is not uncommon for some bariatric surgeons to remove the gallbladder in high-risk patients at the time of their weight loss surgery.*

INCIDENTAL GALLSTONES

> *Question: I had an ultrasound for kidney related issues and was found to have gallstones. What does it mean? Do I need to have my gallbladder taken out? My doctor and I don't think that I have any pain or symptoms related to gallstones.*
>
> *Answer: What you are describing is an incidental finding of gallstones. If you have no symptoms at all, the presence of gallstones does not warrant surgery. Perhaps, it is a wake-up call to eat healthier. Otherwise, no further action is needed from you or your doctor.*

Of patients with incidental gallstones, only 15-25% will end up developing symptoms.

CHAPTER 7

Cholecystitis

Scenario:

Joaquin is a 33-year-old male, who has been having vague abdominal pains in the last few months. Often, these pains would follow mealtimes, but sometimes, they would start out of the blue. He has no other medical problems, but both his mother and grandmother had their gallbladder out before the age of 50. He woke up today with an unrelenting pain in his whole abdomen that is the worst in the upper abdomen. He has experienced some fever and chills, started getting sweaty, and vomited several times. His wife called 911.

In the ER his bloodwork was remarkable for an elevated white count (measurement of infection / inflammation in the blood). On an ultrasound the gallbladder was dilated and swollen, filled with stones, consistent with an infected and inflamed gallbladder.

He was given intravenous antibiotics and fluids in the ER and admitted to the surgical floor. He underwent an uneventful laparoscopic cholecystectomy in the morning.

The condition of INFECTED GALLBLADDER with STONES is called CHOLECYSTITIS.

The symptoms of cholecystitis may include all the symptoms of the biliary colic, such as the following:

Right upper abdominal pain
Pain in Right shoulder blade
Mid upper abdominal pain
Nausea and vomiting

AND some or all symptoms below:

Fever/ chills
Elevated heart rate
Elevated white cell count (WBC) (Elevated WBC represents infection and inflammation in the blood)
Low blood pressure
Confusion
Sepsis

With severe cholecystitis, patient may present in a septic shock (It is rare and seen more in the elderly and immune-suppressed patients).

How is Cholecystitis Clinically Different from Biliary Colic?

While biliary colic is considered a non-surgical condition with no sense of urgency, cholecystitis is in a different ballpark. The presentation of cholecystitis may range from an isolated infection of GB to a full-blown septic shock leading to a shutdown of other organ systems.

Patients with cholecystitis are usually admitted to the surgery floor, but intravenous hydration and antibiotics are started earlier during their workup by the ER staff.

Meanwhile, the surgery team is consulted regarding the admission and scheduling of the surgery.

Most commonly, the surgery is done within 1-3 days of the hospital admission.

Chronic cholecystitis is not uncommon. It may be asymptomatic in people with high pain tolerance. In most, however, it presents with non-specific symptoms that may include occasional fever / chills, pain in the right shoulder blade, vague generalized abdominal pain, left sided abdominal pain, chronic backache, occasional or chronic nausea and vomiting, changes in stool patterns and color, and more.

Scenario:

62-year-old Mary has been having a backache for several years. She would rate it as 3 on a common medical pain severity scale

(The range of this pain scale is 0-10 with 10 being the most unbearable pain, and 0 indicating lack of pain). She brought it up to her primary care doctor (PCP), who initiated a workup. The pain has been present almost daily, and has not been debilitating, but has affected Mary's quality of life, as she has not been able to participate in certain activities with her grandchildren due to it. Mary underwent extensive imaging of the back, including plain X-rays, CT scan and MRI of the thoracic spine, where the pain has been localized. The pain had no correlation with food, so most of her workup was geared towards orthopedic issues. All these studies were essentially normal, except for minor age-related variations.

One day she drove herself to the ER due to exacerbation of the backache, which she rated as 10. In the ER she had labs that showed elevated white cell count. Her x-rays of the back were unremarkable and consistent with normal aging, as before. Her ECG was normal, without any evidence of heart problems. A CAT scan was ordered to find the source of her pain and infection. She was found to have an enlarged, very thickened and swollen gallbladder, filled with hundredths of stones, and with a lot of fluid around the gallbladder.

She was started on intravenous antibiotics and fluids.

She was taken to the operating room the next day, where she was found to have presentation of both acute and chronic cholecystitis. Her gallbladder was "cemented" into the liver, making the surgery extremely difficult. Unfortunately, a complete removal of the gallbladder was not feasible, and subtotal (partial) cholecystectomy was done, along with the placement of a drain next to the remnant of the gallbladder. Her surgery took 3 hours. She stayed several days at the hospital, as she continued to be septic and required intravenous antibiotics. Eventually, she got better, and was discharged home with the drain that was removed later during her ambulatory appointment with her surgeon. Subsequently, she underwent a completion cholecystectomy at a different date, when the rest of the gallbladder was removed.

After the second surgery Mary realized that the backache that was taunting her for years, has disappeared.

There are several interesting points about this case:

The first one is an atypical presentation of the gallbladder disease. Chronic cholecystitis is not something we think of, when patient complains of a backache. The difficulty in diagnosing an atypical presentation of the gallbladder disease can significantly affect patient's quality of life and even survival in some cases.

The other point is the degree of the gallbladder infection that makes it unsafe for the surgeon to remove it completely. In this situation giving up is a sign of wisdom and speaks highly of the surgeon's professional judgement.

Subtotal (partial) cholecystectomy is only performed in the cases of severe cholecystitis, where the removal of the whole gallbladder may be dangerous and result in severe life-threatening complications.

Completion cholecystectomy is usually performed later, when there is no acute infection, and the chronic infection / inflammation of the remaining gallbladder and surrounding areas, has "cooled off".

CHAPTER 8

How is the Gallbladder Disease Diagnosed? Bloodwork and Imaging

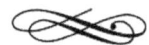

LABS

The lab work for evaluation of the gallbladder disease includes the level of infection in the blood (white cell count or WBC), in addition to the liver enzymes.

Usually, values for kidney function and urine composition are checked, as well.

Liver enzymes are very important in the diagnosis of GB disease.

In the presence of a significant GB infection, the adjacent component of the liver becomes inflamed and infected. This may lead to an elevation of the liver enzymes, such as alkaline phosphatase, aspartate aminotransferase (AST), alanine transaminase (ALT) and total bilirubin.

Additionally, an elevation of liver enzymes may indicate obstruction of bile outflow. This may imply that some gallstones migrated outside the gallbladder, and partially or completely obstructed another duct, such as the common bile duct, for example.

The pancreatic enzymes, such as amylase and lipase, are also obtained to assess for the presence of pancreatitis.

IMAGING

The best initial imaging test for the gallbladder disease is an ultrasound study. It shows the presence or absence of gallstones, along with the characteristics of the gallbladder itself: is GB inflamed / infected? Is it swollen and enlarged?

Other imaging modalities include CAT or CT (Computerized Tomography) MRI (Magnetic Resonance Imaging), and HIDA (Hepatobiliary Iminoacetic Acid).

Of the above, MRI is the most expensive and the most sensitive study for the gallbladder and biliary structures. The MRI that is geared towards biliary system is called MRCP (Magnetic Resonance Cholangiopancreatography).

The CT scan is helpful, but not as sensitive, as the MRCP. It is, however, cheaper and widely available, and allows visualization of other abdominal organs. That gives it a significant diagnostic advantage.

CHAPTER 9

Surgery for Gallbladder Removal: Cholecystectomy

Laparoscopic cholecystectomy (LC) is the standard in the Western world.

It is performed under general anesthesia, meaning the patient is put to sleep during the surgery, and breathes with the help of the ventilator.

This laparoscopic procedure is considered a major surgery.

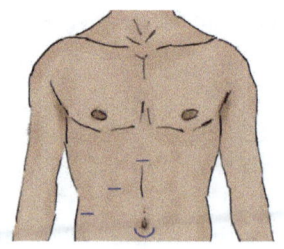

Laparoscopic Cholecystectomy Incisions

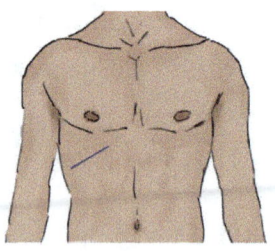

Open Cholecystectomy Incision

The advantages of LC include shorter hospital stays, less postoperative pain, better cosmetic appearance, and quicker return to work.

Once the patient is comfortably sedated and connected to the ventilator, the surgery is started with an incision in or below the belly button. A hollow short pipe-like device, called a trocar, is placed into the incision. Then a special tubing is attached to this device, and gas is insufflated through it into the abdomen. The abdomen becomes very bloated and taut. Then 2 or 3 incisions are made, and the other trocars are placed. The surgical instruments are placed into the abdomen through these trocars.

If GB is very infected, then inflammation and scarring may obscure GB visualization, and it may take some time for the surgeon to clean / dissect GB and adjacent portion of the liver. The main steps of this procedure include the following:

The surgeon identifies the whole gallbladder, and focuses on the cystic duct / gallbladder transition

Both the cystic duct and artery are identified, and the surgeon starts placing the clips using a stapler-like device for an anticipated transection of each of these structures.

Both the cystic duct and cystic artery are transected in the areas defined by the clips, thus freeing the gallbladder from these important connections.

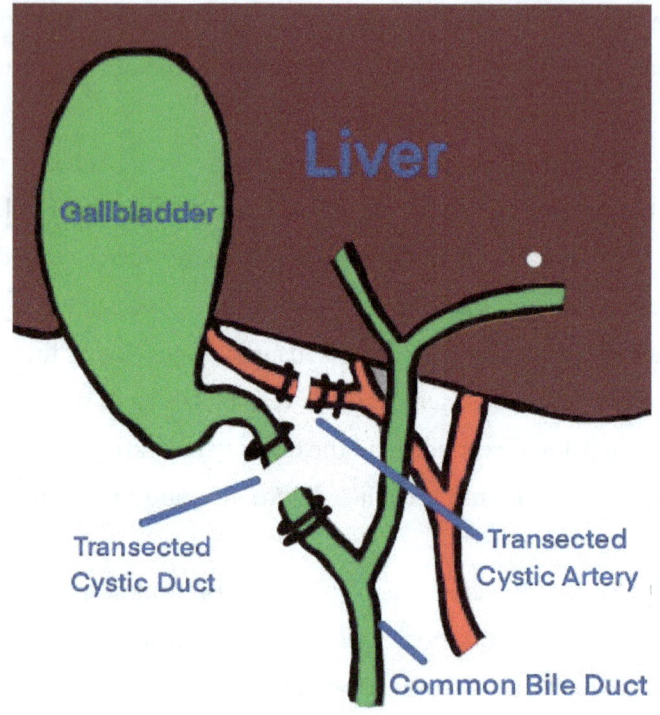

The gallbladder is then dissected / peeled off the liver bed. The free gallbladder is now removed via the largest trocar, often in a special plastic bag.

The trocars are taken out, and incisions are closed.

It is very important to get the air out of the abdomen before closing the incisions.

Any leftover air would irritate the diaphragm and result into post-operative right shoulder pain.

The incisions are closed with invisible absorbable sutures. The patient is woken up and taken to post-operative area.

CHAPTER 10

What Can Go Wrong? Risks and Complications

As much as we don't want to think about adverse reactions and complications of the surgery, unfortunately, LC has its own risks.

The surgery may take anywhere from 15 min to 3+ hours (Rare).

Why? The duration of the surgery is directly proportional to the level

of inflammation, infection and scarring of the diseased gallbladder.

The goal is to correctly identify and visualize all the structures, especially the cystic duct and cystic artery, before cutting them. Many scientific papers have been written about the exact steps / algorithms to streamline this crucial step. LC is a surgery where the lack of attention to details may lead to a devastating complication, or even death. The reason is the location of the gallbladder that is in close proximity of important organs (bowel, liver), ducts and blood vessels.

Laparoscopic cholecystectomy is often called a $100 surgery with a million-dollar cost, if there is a complication. It is because a surgeon's reimbursement for this surgery is low (no, not $100, but not too far from it), but potential complications could be devastating in both medical and legal fees. Since this surgery is so frequently performed, and 95% of the time it goes very well, its complexity is often underestimated by non-surgical doctors, who often describe it as a "piece of cake".

The role of a surgeon is to give patients confidence in a good outcome, and yet be able to inform them of potential complications.

The list of complications includes, but not limited to:

1) Injury to biliary ducts, especially the Common Bile Duct (CBD)
This dreaded injury has 5% occurrence. Injury to CBD is usually managed by another surgery, requiring drains, and often a repeat surgery. In short, the consequences of CBD injury may be devastating.

2) Injuries to blood vessels: Bleeding may range from minor oozing to a major bleed. Ultimately, life-threatening bleeding may occur.

3) Injury to liver: It may vary from a minor abrasion to a deep laceration with the latter having the worst outcomes.

4) Injury to bowel, diaphragm: these injuries are very serious, and would require a return to the operating room for another surgery to repair the issue.

5) Bile Leak from the cystic duct stump: this happens when the clips on the remnant of the cystic duct migrate, or completely fall off, and bile starts leaking out. This is a relatively minor injury that could be remedied without a repeat surgery.

6) Retained bile duct stones: this could be fixed with stone removal via endoscopic (through mouth) procedure called ERCP

7) Spillage of stones: this may occur when gallbladder is very infected, dilated and inflamed. Manipulation of gallbladder may result in its perforation and resulting spillage of the stones into the abdominal cavity. These stones are likely to show on imaging, especially, if they are calcium stones.

These stones may be asymptomatic or may lead to an infection and even abscesses.

CHAPTER 11

What Happens After Surgery? Post-Operative Course

After an uneventful laparoscopic cholecystectomy, the patient may be discharged home the next day, or even later the same day, if the surgery took place in the morning.

The patient is advised to avoid heavy lifting for 6 weeks to prevent development of a hernia in the umbilical incision.

The patient is encouraged to take over-the-counter pain medications, such as Tylenol and Ibuprofen, unless they are allergic to them. Opioid pain medications are given to be taken for breakthrough pain.

It is important to note that patient should not be driving or working while taking narcotics.

Most people end up taking narcotics for 1-2 days. That is one of the advantages of laparoscopic surgery, as it leads to much milder post-operative pain, that can be managed at home.

One of the commonly reported symptoms after the surgery is pain in the shoulder, usually on the right side. It is attributed to irritation of the diaphragm by the air that was insufflated during the procedure.

Although the surgeon lets the air out of the abdomen in the end of surgery / before closing the incisions, there is often some residual air left.

It goes away by itself within the next few weeks.

CHAPTER 12

What Really Happens with the GI System After Cholecystectomy?

Diarrhea is the most common post-surgery issue!

Approximately 50% of patients experience change in their bowel habits after the surgery. The change is usually a new onset of diarrhea and bowel urgency.
In most patients (77%), it resolves after 6 months.
Traditionally, a low-fat diet was recommended after gallbladder removal.

Recent study from Spain has shown that a low-fat diet does not seem to affect or improve diarrhea after cholecystectomy.
This implies that either our GI system adapts to the absence of the gallbladder with time by normalizing the bowel movements; or, perhaps, there is another factor that regulates this, that has not been discovered yet.

It is also not unusual to see a weight gain after surgery, as there is no longer pain after eating that would stop the person from eating high-fat foods.

CHAPTER 13

Diet After Gallbladder Surgery

Strictly speaking, adhering to low-fat diet is a good idea after any intestinal surgery.

During any surgery that involves GI tract: large and small intestine, gallbladder, stomach, etc., the GI tract slows down.

It is a natural response to trauma. Yes, any surgery is a trauma to a human body, even though it is curative.

Just like when time slows down when we are in shock or experiencing something scary, the intestinal motility slows down, and in some cases even shuts down after the surgery.

In these rare cases the patient is unable to pass gas and have a bowel movement, and this condition is called POSTOPERATIVE ILEUS.

The elderly and immune-suppressed patients are more prone to it. With postoperative ileus, the patient is not discharged home, as they are unable to eat. They are kept in the hospital with intravenous hydration; and, sometimes, a nasogastric tube is inserted through the nose to suction air to avoid further bloating and vomiting.

So, eating small frequent low-fat meals after the surgery is a good idea for most, if not all GI surgeries.
That way the body gently eases back into eating.
In children this easing-into process may take a few days.
In elderly patients, it may take 6 weeks or more.

In summary, there are many books written about diet after gallbladder surgery, complete with recipes, however, there is a very minimal scientific data to provide any definitive recommendations.

CHAPTER 14

Special Situations: Choledocholithiasis and Cholangitis or When Gallstones Obstruct Common Bile Duct (CBD)

Choledocholithiasis is the presence of gallstones in CBD, and it occurs in less than 15% of patients younger than 60 years of age, and in 60% of elderly patients.

The risk factors for choledocholithiasis are like the ones for cholelithiasis, except for some prevalence in males and in the elderly.

CBD that is obstructed with stones, may appear dilated on an ultrasound, but that is not always true. CBD may appear completely normal, and, additionally, the CBD stones may not be visible on an ultrasound.

When presence of CBD stones is suspected, an MRI study called MRCP is obtained.

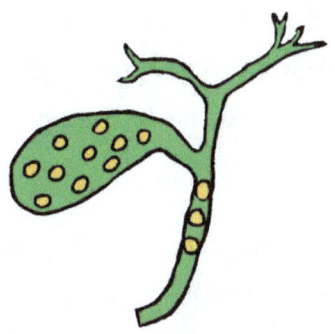

Choledocholithiasis

Scenario:

Michael is a 68-year-old man who lives with his family. He has high blood pressure, high cholesterol, and gout. He is of average weight. His family noticed that the whites of his eyes were becoming yellow, and his skin started taking on bronze hue, although he had not been tanning. He noted some vague discomfort throughout his upper abdomen in the last 2 months or so. He lost about 5 lbs.

This time the episode became more intense, with the pain being steady and unrelenting. He also felt a little warm but did not have a thermometer to check his temperature.

After 5 hours of this pain, he decided to drive himself to the ER.

In the ER he was found to have an elevated white blood cell count (WBC), and significantly elevated liver enzymes. His ultrasound showed a swollen and thickened gallbladder that was filled with gallstones. His CBD appeared a little dilated. MRCP was obtained and showed several obstructing stones in the CBD. Surgery and GI teams were called. GI team started evaluating the patient for ERCP.

ERCP=endoscopic retrograde cholangiopancreatography (Thank God for abbreviations!)

ERCP is somewhat an invasive test that combines endoscopy and X-ray techniques. Endoscopy involves an insertion of a thin tube (endoscope) through the mouth into stomach and small intestine. The X-ray part entails injection of a dye through the catheter to visualize biliary structures, pancreatic ducts and pancreas while performing an X-ray at the same time.
Although ERCP is mostly safe, there are risks associated with it, such as bleeding, infection, perforation of ducts, and inflammation of pancreas.
This procedure is done under general anesthesia.

ERCP is very helpful not only in identifying the stones in the ducts, but also in treating / removing them. In fact, ERCP obliterated the complex and potentially life-threatening open surgeries that were done in the past to accomplish the same. ERCP is utilized for stone retrieval with the help of special extraction balloons or baskets.

Following ERCP, cholecystectomy is still recommended. It could be done during the same admission (usually recommended), or later.

Back to our patient, Michael:

He underwent ERCP with successful retrieval of the stones from CBD. He had laparoscopic cholecystectomy the next day and went home the day after.

Obstruction of the common bile duct with stones may lead to the infection of CBD, that is called CHOLANGITIS.

Cholangitis presents as jaundice, fever, chills, abdominal pain (more right sided, but not always), nausea / vomiting, light colored stools, dark urine. If untreated, cholangitis will lead to full body infection (sepsis) with a very high mortality rate. That is why decompression (removal) of obstructing stones from CBD is an utmost priority.

CHAPTER 15

Special Situations: Gallstone Pancreatitis or When Gallstones Obstruct Pancreas

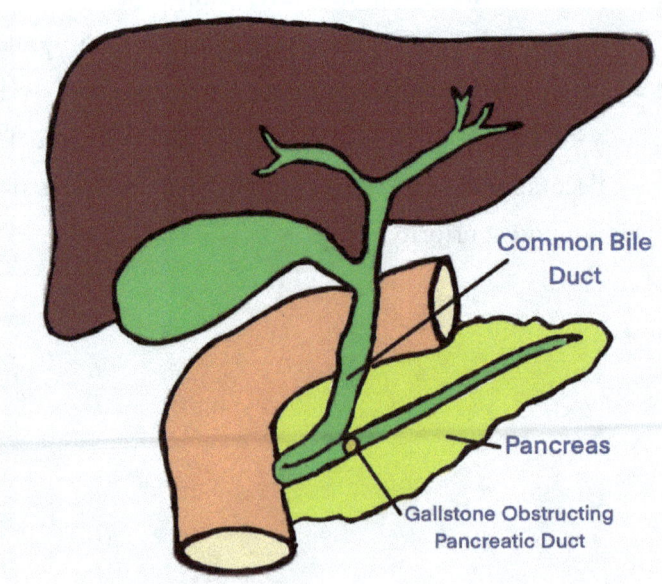

Gallstones often are the cause of pancreatitis. Small stones may induce it by blocking a pancreatic duct, and thus causing inflammation and even infection of the pancreas.

Alternatively, blockage of an opening in the 1st part of the small intestine, called duodenum, will lead to pancreatitis, as well.

The initial goal in the treatment of gallstone pancreatitis is to remove the stones via ERCP. However, the treatment of gallstone pancreatitis is not that simplistic, and, rather, multifactorial.

Performing ERCP in patients with pancreatitis may exacerbate pancreatitis, despite the removal of the initial offending agent (gallstones). Pancreatitis may be mild and then escalate to sepsis and, unfortunately, death. Thus, even the mildest form of pancreatitis is taken seriously.

Patients with moderate pancreatitis are often kept in the Intensive Care Unit (ICU) for continuous monitoring, intravenous hydration and proximity of life-saving care, if the need arises.

Recovery from gallstone pancreatitis means that the patient is stable, pain-free and their pancreatic enzymes are normal or almost normal. At that point laparoscopic cholecystectomy should be performed.

CHAPTER 16

Special Situations: Gallstone Ileus or When Gallstones Obstruct Small Bowel

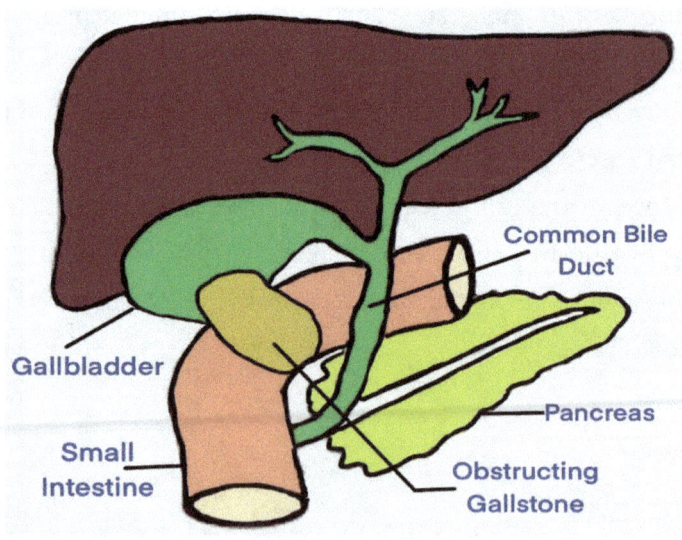

Gallstone Ileus is an uncommon manifestation of gallstones. In this case the stone erodes through the wall of the gallbladder into the intestine.

Usually, it is the small intestine, but, rarely, stomach or colon may be involved. This abnormal connection between the two organs that is reinforced by the stone is called cholecysto-enteric fistula. For a stone to cause an obstruction it must be quite large, at least 2 cm in diameter.

The symptoms of gallstone ileus are bloating, constipation, inability to pass gas, nausea and vomiting. The dreaded complication of this condition is peritonitis, when there is a perforation of the intestine from an obstruction, along with the resulting spillage of stool into the abdominal cavity.

When a patient presents with gallstone ileus, first a nasogastric tube is inserted through the nose to decompress air and bile. Subsequently, patient is rushed to the operating room for an emergent laparotomy or laparoscopic exploration. The first step is to remove the stone by making an incision in the affected part of the intestine. If intestine looks healthy, the hole through which the stone is removed, is repaired (sutured).

If any part of the affected intestine is not viable, then removal of this section of the intestine must be done. The decision to remove the gallbladder at the same time is more complex. It depends on the stability of the patient, the state of gallbladder infection / inflammation, and, in general, the degree of frailty of the patient. Since this rare condition often occurs in patients with many other medical issues, often removal of the gallbladder at the time of stone removal / intestinal repair or resection, may not be safe. The gallbladder is removed later, and sometimes, not removed at all, if the patient is at a very high risk for the subsequent surgery.

CHAPTER 17

Special Situations: Gallbladder Disease When There Are No Gallstones at all

Acalculous cholecystitis is an infection of the gallbladder in the absence of stones.

This condition is not very common, and usually is seen in the elderly and immune-compromised patients, especially, when they are hospitalized for other issues. It may present as a swollen and dilated gallbladder, accompanied by the right-sided abdominal pain. Most frequently, there are components of gallbladder necrosis and infection that may lead to gallbladder perforation, gangrene and, ultimately, peritonitis (infection of the whole abdominal cavity) and sepsis.

In the case of frank perforation and peritonitis, surgery is lifesaving.

However, since these patients are already very debilitated, the stress of the surgery, including general anesthesia, may be extremely straining by itself. So, unless surgery is the only solution, such as in the case of peritonitis, a percutaneous cholecystostomy presents a safer and less invasive solution.

It entails a placement of the thin plastic tube under X-ray (ultrasound or CT- guidance). The tube drains the infected bile and decompresses the gallbladder. Along with intravenous antibiotics, it is a great temporary measure. It is temporary, as ultimately, the gallbladder still needs to be removed.

However, if patient continues to be a suboptimal candidate for surgery, then the cholecystostomy tube may be removed in a few weeks without definitive plans for a future surgery. By that time, the patient is usually at the rehab or in the nursing home or, less commonly, at home.

Although, it is not the most pleasant experience, the presence of this drain doesn't stop one from performing daily activities. The drain is sutured to the skin, and there is a plastic container at the end to collect the drainage. Usually, the drain is tucked under the outer clothing, and needs to be emptied periodically, depending on the amount of drainage. Patients themselves could perform this simple task.

Removal of the drain entails a crude, and, unfortunately, painful pulling that lasts a few seconds. It is performed during an outpatient visit with the surgeon.

GALLBLADDER DISEASE

Scenario:

John is an 85-year-old male with heart disease, high blood pressure, thyroid issues, diabetes, and gout.

He lives at a nursing home. His family lives out of state. He woke up confused and disoriented with a fever of 101.8, clutching his abdomen. One of the aides noted that his abdomen was bloated. Per nursing home records, he had not complained of any abdominal pain, and always had a good appetite. He vomited, and then collapsed. 911 was called, and the patient was eventually admitted to the ICU.

He had a CAT scan and a subsequent ultrasound of his abdomen that showed an enlarged, dilated and very thickened gallbladder with no stones, but with a lot of fluid around the gallbladder.

John was found to be septic with low blood pressure and elevated level of infection in the blood. Additionally, his blood cultures showed Klebsiella and E.coli (two bacteria that live in the GI tract). In the ICU he was started on intravenous antibiotics, and blood pressure enhancing medications, as he was in shock, and his blood pressure continued to be very low. He also had a urinary catheter and nasogastric tube inserted. Subsequently, he was found to be in a multi-organ failure with the decrease in functionality of cardiac, respiratory and renal *systems. He had to be intubated and was placed on the ventilator. A cholecystostomy tube was placed urgently.*

After 2 weeks in the ICU, he was able to come off the ventilator, as his condition stabilized. He went to the rehab after one month in the hospital. His cholecystostomy tube was removed 8 weeks after its placement. At that time there was a clear bile output with no more pus noted. Laparoscopic cholecystectomy was offered to him, but it was explained to him and his family that he was at a high risk for intra and post-operative complications. Patient declined the surgery, and incidentally, he never had another bout of cholecystitis.

CHAPTER 18

Special Situations: Slow Gallbladder

There is a condition called gallbladder dyskinesia, which essentially constitutes a lazy or, rather, overwhelmed gallbladder.

It presents as pain in right abdomen that may or may not follow meals. Other symptoms, such as nausea, vomiting and bloating may be present, as well. This functional disorder is suspected when patient has biliary colic-like pains without presence of gallstones or any lab or ultrasound abnormalities. There is a test to check the efficiency of the gallbladder function. As you recall, the gallbladder must eject bile in response to fatty meals. HIDA (Hepatobiliary Iminoacetic Acid) scan is a study that measures this efficiency.

During this test a radioactive tracer is injected intravenously. This tracer then becomes part of bile formation and ejection. The propagation of the tracer is tracked via imaging. The imaging may take hours to produce results. The more sluggish is the gallbladder, the longer it will take for the tracker to propagate. The number that gets measured is the ejection fraction (EF) of the gallbladder. The EF of less than 40% is considered indicative of a dysfunctional gallbladder. The presence of biliary colic-like pains and low gallbladder EF qualify the patient for laparoscopic cholecystectomy.

CHAPTER 19

Growths in Gallbladder

POLYPS

Polyps are growths in the gallbladder wall. They could be non-neoplastic and neoplastic. Non-neoplastic polyps are benign. Most of them are made of cholesterol, and a small fraction of them is inflammatory.

Neoplastic polyps mostly comprised of adenomas. Adenomas need to be monitored with an ultrasound for any increase in size. The possibility of their malignant transformation starts increasing with further growth. If the polyp is getting to be 10 mm or more, then surgery is indicated.

GALLBLADDER CANCER

This cancer is very rare, but, unfortunately, often fatal. It is frequently diagnosed while the patient is undergoing laparoscopic cholecystectomy due to gallstones. Often, it is too late to achieve a cure, as the cancer is far too advanced.

Some factors that predispose to gallbladder cancer are smoking, female gender, obesity, advanced age, presence of gallstones, abnormal bile duct anatomy, history of typhoid infection due to Salmonella.

The treatment for gallbladder cancer depends on how far it has spread. In many cases, by the time gallbladder cancer is diagnosed, it has already metastasized to adjacent lymph nodes and to other organs. That makes it usually inoperable. If surgery is feasible, usually a portion of the adjacent liver is removed, along with the gallbladder and the lymph nodes.

Conclusion

The gallbladder is a small, but fascinating organ. One can survive and live well without it. Despite being one of the most common diseases seen in the emergency department, its diagnosis and treatment are not always straightforward.

It is noteworthy that at the present time there is no definitive way to treat advanced diseases of the gallbladder without removing it.

As in many gastrointestinal conditions, in the absence of genetic factors, healthy diet is the only preventative and protective measure for the diseases of the gallbladder.

References

Articles

Di Ciaula A, Wang DQH, Portincasa P. An Update on the pathogenesis of cholesterol gallstone disease. Curr Opin Gastroenterol. 2018 Mar; 34(2): 71-80

Lam R, Zakko A, Petrov JC, Kumar P, Duffy AJ, Muniraj T. Gallbladder disorders: a comprehensive review. Dis. Mon. 2021 July;67(7):101130

Soloway RD, Trotman BW, Ostrow JD. Pigment Gallstones. Gastroenterology. 1977 Jan;72(1):167-82

Trotman BW. Pigment gallstone disease. Gastroenterol Clin North Am. 1991 Mar;20(1):111-26

Blasco YR, Munante MP, Gomez-Fernandez L, Jovell-Fernandez E, Oms Bernad LM. Low- fat diet after cholecystectomy: Should it be systematically recommended? Cir Esp (Engl Ed). 2020 Jan;98(1):36-42

Simon M, Hassan IN, Ramasamy D, Wilson D. Primary choledocolithiasis 15 years postcholecystectomy. Case Rep Med. 2020 Published online 2020 Oct 26

Zakko SF, Overview of gallstone disease in adults. In: UpToDate, Chopra S (Ed), UpToDate, Apr 25, 2022

Books
Hassler KR, Collins JT, Philip K, Jones MW. Laparoscopic Cholecystectomy
2022 Apr 13

About the Author

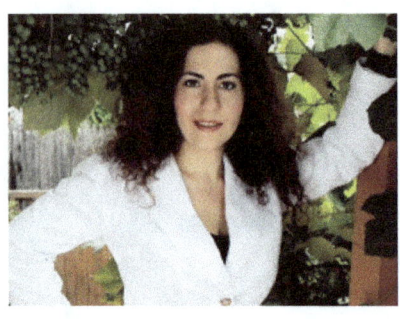

Dr. Azizian is a board-certified general surgeon, licensed in the states of Massachusetts, Vermont, and New Hampshire. In addition to performing surgeries, Dr. Azizian takes great joy in educating her patients. A large component of her daily life is spent on explaining medical concepts to her patients in an easy-to-understand manner.

As an educator, she is often invited to speak on various medical topics.

Dr. Azizian's interest in medical education stems from her belief that being educated about their health helps patients make a truly informed decision about their medical care.

Dr. Azizian resides in Massachusetts with her husband and three children.

www.ingramcontent.com/pod-product-compliance
Lightning Source LLC
Chambersburg PA
CBHW051538240526
45465CB00027B/716